Disclaimer

I0494146

This book is intended to be a general guide, to raise awareness, and to help people make informed decisions in the context of their own personal circumstance.

As everybody's circumstances are different, so are the remedies you should seek. While many of the remedies in this book can be applied by almost anybody regardless of their conditions, they are not intended and should not be relied upon to replace personal medical advice.

The author accepts no responsibility for any loss, be it personal or financial, as a result for the use or misuse of the information in this book.

If you have any doubts or concerns after reading this book, please speak to a doctor or other qualified person before taking any actions.

INTRODUCTION

Essential oils are the highly concentrated liquids extracted from stems, flowers, leaves or parts of various plants. The essential oil, through its chemical properties, is capable of providing physical and psychological benefits as it revitalises many of the body's natural systems by carrying nutrients and oxygen to the cells. Benefits includes improvements of mental clarity, stress relief, cold & flu relief, skin care treatments and hair care treatments.

Essential oil is one natural healing liquid that is completely holistic as it works not only around the physical sphere, to make people look good, but also flourishes their emotional and mental grounds to make them holistically content.

This book is of the awareness that essential oil molecules contain compounds which can cross the blood train barrier and enter the brain thereby contributing to immense improvement of mental clarity. This book is all about the important things you need to know about essential oil as well as the best options you have with essential oil. This book can be a starting point that can lead you towards taking active decisions as regards using a natural alternative to cough syrups, pain medications and decongestants to treat symptoms of cold and flues.

Contents

Chapter 1

What Are Essential Oils?

Essential oils are the highly concentrated liquid extracted from stems, flowers, leaves or other parts of various plants. This liquid is usually distilled into a pure oil.
Essential oils are not actually oils, but are called oils because they are usually slippery and are not usually water soluble. Essential oils are also known volatile oils because they will evaporate into the air.
Most essential oils are clear, however some oils, such as citrus oils, may have a yellow or amber tinge to them. Sometimes, the colour of an oil is a good indication of it's purity.
Five of the must have essential oils are:
1. Frankincense
2. Peppermint
3. Eucalyptus
4. Lemon-grass
5. Lavender

Each essential oil has its own chemical properties that are capable of providing physical and psychological benefits.

Just because essential oils have a strong odour, don't confuse them with fragrance or perfumed oils. Synthetic fragrance oils do not offer the same medicinal or therapeutic benefits as plant-based essential oils.

Depending on the application, essential oils can be inhaled in various ways. Diluted oil may be applied to the skin, and depending on the desired effect, may be blended with other ingredients.

The four most common personal uses for essential oils include:

1. Aromatherapy
2. Massage therapy
3. Lotions
4. Natural remedies

Some other uses for essential oils which are beyond the scope of this book include:

- Candles
- Ingredients for home-made cleaning products
- Bath salts
- Pet products
- Insect control products

Eleven important things you need to know about essential oils

1. **Essential oil molecules are microscopic in size-** Because essential oil molecules are so small, they are readily absorbed into the skin which makes them ideal for lotions and other personal care items meant to heal, soothe and nourish.

2. **Most essential oils should not be applied undiluted to your skin-** Because they are so concentrated, if essential oils are to be used directly on the skin, they first need to be diluted. Various substances may be used to dilute them including butter, alcohol or various natural "real" oils such as olive or jojoba. Failure to dilute essential oils may result in an unforeseen reaction.

3. **Never use undiluted oil on a child or baby- Children** have more delicate skin than adults and are therefore much more sensitive to it than adults. If you intend to use an essential oil recipe on a child make sure you only use half the amount of essential oil recommended in the recipe.

4. **Never leave essential oils within the reach of children- Essential** oils can be hazardous if left unattended in small hands.

5. **Never internally consume essential oils-** There are no proven benefits to internally consuming essential oils and some of them may be harmful if taken internally.

6. **Know what you're allergic to-** Before using essential oils, make sure you are familiar with any allergies you may have; for example, if you are allergic to rosemary or oregano, you will also be allergic to their essential oils.

7. **Essential oils should be stored in dark containers-** Direct exposure to sunlight will deteriorate the quality of essential oils, so make sure you store them in a dark container in a dark place to insure you get the longest possible shelf life out of your oils.

8. **A simple test to help determine the purity of essential oils-** The easiest way to test the purity of many store bought oils is to place a drop of oil in a piece of paper. If the oil quickly evaporates leaving no ring behind, then this is a good indication that the oil is pure. If the oil does not evaporate quickly and/or a ring is left behind, then this is a good indication that the essential oil has been mixed with some sort or "real" oil.

9. **A simple test to see if you're sensitive to a particular oil before you start using it-** Mix a drop of the particular essential oil you intend to use with a half a teaspoon of olive or jojoba oil. Apply this mixture to the inner, upper part of your arm and wait a few hours. If no redness or irritation occurs it is most likely that you are safe to use this oil.

10. **Most essential oils can be stored for a very long time-** If you are wondering if you should purchase an essential oil you rarely use, it might be worth noting that if properly stored, most essential oils will retain their effectiveness for up to ten years.

11. **Avoid using essential oils when pregnant-** Some compounds in many essential oils may behave similarly to hormones due to their molecular structure, so it is recommended that you avoid using essential oils during pregnancy, especially during the first trimester.

Chapter 2

How To Use Essential Oils To Improve Your Mental Clarity

The three subjects have been included in this chapter because the simplest and easiest way to use essential oils to improve your mental clarity is to vaporise and inhale the oil vapours, and the two methods for doing this are:

The Candle Oil Defuser Method

A candle oil defuser can be bought very affordably at many discount stores and is great for defusing essential oils for a multitude of uses.
They are great at night time in a sealed room.
Just make sure you don't let children or pets near them unsupervised, or use them near any fire hazard.

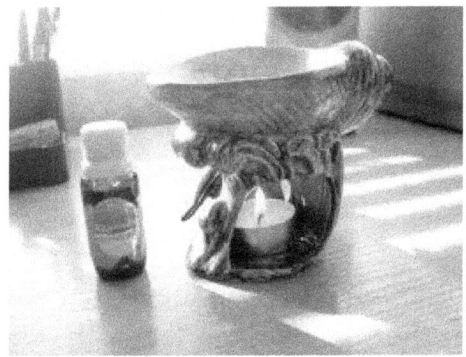

Above: A candle essential oil defuser.
The Hot Water Method

Possibly the easiest and simplest way to vaporise your essential oils is to simply drop your oils into a pot with a little boiling water on your stove.
Add the oil as the water in the pot starts to steam and turn the heat down.

Essential oils can revitalise many of the body's natural systems by carrying nutrients and oxygen to the cells.
Essential oil molecules contain compounds which can cross the blood train barrier and enter the brain.
Research suggests that essential oils may be useful for cleansing heavy metals such as aluminium that lodge in the brain and contribute to Alzheimer's disease and memory loss.
They can also target parts of the brain related to emotion and that store pleasure and trauma.

Five main essential oils which improve mental clarity include:

1. Basil oil.
2. Rosemary oil.
3. Juniper berry oil.
4. Sage oil.
5. Peppermint oil.

Any of these oils can be used on their own to help improve mental clarity or they can be blended with other essential oils.

Here are two simple blends you can use to help improve your mental clarity:

Recipe 1

1. 6 drops of eucalyptus oil.
2. 5 drops of basil oil.
3. 2 drops of peppermint oil.

Recipe 2

1. 3 drops of sage oil.
2. 4 drops of juniper berry oil.
3. 3 drops of rosemary oil.

How To Use Essential Oils For Stress Relief

The amygdala is a small part located within the temporal lobes of the brain and forms part of the brain's limbic system. The amygdala plays an important role in modulating stress response in the brain especially where feelings of anxiety and fear are concerned.
Essential oils can effect the limbic system and therefore can be used for stress relief.

Five essential oils which have been proven to help combat stress include:

1. Frankincense oil.
2. Lavender oil.
3. Jasmine oil.
4. Bergamot oil.
5. Grapefruit oil.
6. Geranium oil.

Any of these oils can help reduce stress, however here are two blends you might like to try. As in the previous chapter, the simplest and quickest method to use these oils is to vaporise them and inhale them using the techniques outlined earlier in this chapter.

Recipe 1

1. 1 drop of lemon oil.
2. 3 drops of sage oil.
3. 1 drop of lavender oil.

Recipe 2

1. 1 drop of frankincense oil.
2. 3 drops of bergamot oil.
3. 1 drop of geranium oil.

Chapter 3

How To Use Essential Oils For Cold & Flu Relief

While there are many different cough syrups, pain medications and decongestants on the market today, many people are looking for more natural alternatives to treat the symptoms of cold and flu, and while essential oils will never take the place of a proper consultation from a doctor, they can help reduce the discomfort of coughs, congestion and sinus pressure.

Here are some ways you can use essential oils to relieve some of the symptoms of cold and flu.

Cough- Eucalyptus oil is great for clearing congestion of the lungs. Most essential oils derived from leaves are good for relieving congestion from the lungs. To massage the chest in a six ounce bottle, mix ten drops of bergamot, ten drops of lemon, two drops jojoba, five drops of cedar wood, and ten drops of eucalyptus. After you have rubbed your chest, you can inhale the essential oil residue on your hands by cupping your hands over you nose and breathing in.

Fever- Add three drops of lavender, one drop of peppermint and one cup of ice cold water to a bowl. Mix the solution well and immerse a wash cloth into the solution. Wring out the wash cloth and place it on the forehead. Repeat this process several times and replace the water when it has reached room temperature.

Congestion of the sinuses- Combine two drops of jojoba, five drops of green tea oil, five drops of peppermint oil, twenty drops of lavender oil and five drops of eucalyptus oil in a six ounce bottle. Avoiding the eyes, massage this decongestant blend on your face, paying particular attention to the upper lip, and make sure you inhale as you apply this blend. Alternatively, you can add a capful of this blend to a facial steam or to a bath. This can also be used in a defuser as described in the previous chapter, or to use this as a spray mist, combine this blend with some distilled water in as spray bottle and shake the bottle before spraying.

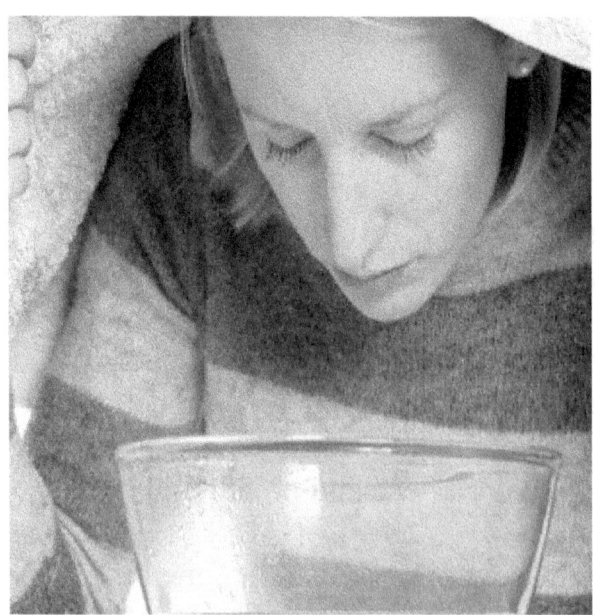

Above: Stream vaporisation is a great way to use essential oils to treat a cold.

Chapter 4

Essential Oil Skin Care Treatments

Essential oils have various therapeutic qualities which enhance any cream, and some oils have specialized qualities which can aid skin conditions.

Many skin care products today contain essential oils, so why not make your own natural skin care products at a fraction of the cost?

Essential Oil Lip Balm

Ingredients

- 1 ½ teaspoons of vitamin E essential oil.
- 2 ounces of cosmetic quality bees wax.
- 1 tablespoon + 2 ounces of extra virgin coconut oil.
- 25 ounces of peppermint or vanilla essential oil.

Method

1. Place the beeswax, coconut oil and vitamin oil into a glass measuring cup.
2. Half fill a pan with water and boil.
3. When the water in the pan is slightly boiling place the glass measuring cup in the pan to melt the bees wax and oil.

4. When you see that every thing has melted mix all the ingredients together to combine them.
5. Pour your lip balm into a clean lip balm jar or other small container.

When the balm has dried and properly solidified you will be able to use your new balm.

Essential Oil Acme Treatment

Ingredients

- 7 drops of tea tree or lemon grass oil.
- 30 ml of jojoba or olive oil (or if you prefer a gel use aloe vera).
- 10 drops of lavender oil.
- 3 drops of geranium.

Method

1. In a dark bottle combine all the above ingredients.
2. Close the bottle and shake well.
3. Making sure you avoid the nose, eyes and lips, use a cotton bud to apply a small amount to the effected skin twice a day.

Moisturising Essential Oil Face Mask

Ingredients

- 2 drops of frankincense oil.
- 2 drops of neroli oil.
- 2 drops of rose oil.
- 6 teaspoons of apricot oil.
- 1 teaspoon of honey.
- Finely ground almond.

Method

1. Combine the oil and the honey in a glass measuring cup.
2. Half fill a pan with water and boil.
3. When the water in the pan is slightly boiling, place the glass measuring cup in the pan to boil.
4. When you see that the honey has melted, gently mix all the ingredients together to combine them.
5. Now, still mixing everything, slowly add the crushed almond till you form a smooth paste.
6. Remove the pan from the heat.
7. Once the mixture has sufficiently cooled, you can apply it to your face.

A Healing Toner For Sensitive Skin

Ingredients

- ¼ cup of rose hydro-sol or rose water.
- 4 drops of rose oil.
- 2 tablespoons of witch hazel.
- 2 drops of yarrow oil.

Method

Combine all the ingredients in a glass bottle and shake well.

Chapter 5

Essential Oil Hair Care Treatments

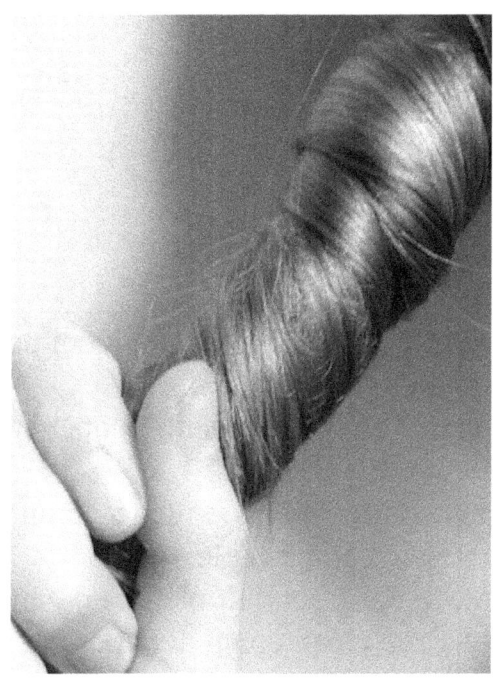

Essential oils can revitalize your hear and scalp. They can be used to improve or treat a variety of ailments including controlling dandruff and scalp irritation, straightening hair, cleansing the scalp and possibly even encourage hair growth. Some essential oils can improve the condition of the hair while others can improve the condition of the scalp.

Below are just some essential oil recipes which can help improve the condition of your hair and scalp.

Essential Oil Talc Shampoo

Ingredients

- 25 grams of pure talcum powder
- 4 drops of tea tree oil
- 4 drops of rosemary oil
- 4 drops of lavender oil

Method

1. Gently place the 25 grams of talcum powder in a blender.
2. Place the lid on the blender and open the small lid in the centre of the large lid.
3. Add the oils drop by drop while running the blender at the slowest speed possible.
4. Now, place the essential oil and talcum blend in a suitably sized clean container and seal it firmly.

How to use

Over a bath or some other place where any excess shampoo can be washed away, using a quality brush, brush about two teaspoons through you hair.
To use the talc shampoo, brush two teaspoons through your hair.

Dry Hair Conditioner Oil

Ingredients

- 3 drops of rosemary oil
- 1 tablespoon of jojoba or canola oil

Method

Using a small bowl, combine the oils and mix.

How to use

1. Using warm water, wet the hair and apply the conditioner.
2. Let the conditioner sit in the hair for twenty minutes.
3. Now, rinse you hair.

Other uses

Scalp Massage

Simply place three drops of conditioner oil on you finger tips and thoroughly massage it into the scalp.

Split End Avocado/Essential Oil Wrap

Ingredients

- 1 Avocado
- 10 drops of almond oil.
- 4 teaspoons of honey

Method

1. Peel and remove the stone from the avocado.
2. Combine all the ingredients in a blender and blend the ingredients until they are thoroughly combined.

How to use

1. Completely massage this mixture into wet hair whilst paying particular attention to the tips of the hair.

2. Wrap the hair in a towel or clear plastic wrap.

3. Leave the wrap on for thirty minutes.

4. Thoroughly rinse the hair with warm water.

Chapter 6

Description Of Each Essential And Carrier Oil Mentioned In This Book

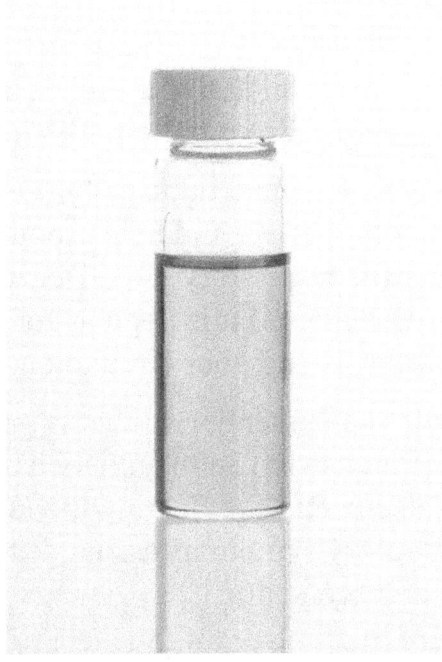

Almond oil- a popular carrier oil and commonly used in aromatherapy, it is suitable for most skin types. It is also commonly used in many baby skin care range of products. Below are some of the benefits of almond oil for the skin.

Apricot- is a carrier oil and is great for mature and dehydrated skin as it works to sooth and moisturise the skin.

Basil oil- is an essential oil and is useful for treating depression and digestive ailments. It is also used as an insecticide and stimulant. It should not be used on children under fifteen years old and expectant mothers.

Bergamot oil- is an essential oil often used to treat stress, tension, and skin ailments such as eczema and psoriasis. It should not be applied to sensitive skin which will be exposed to sun as it may cause burns.

Coconut oil- is a carrier oil and is useful as a skin moisturiser and to help prevent protein loss in hair.

Eucalyptus oil- is an essential oil usually used for colds and fever as it has a cooling effect and helps sooth throat infection and clear the respiratory tract. Because eucalyptus oil also acts as a warming oil it is popular for treating muscular pains, arthritis and poor circulation.

Frankincense oil- is an essential oil that is great for calming the mind and is often used to calm anxiety and for meditation. It is also useful for clearing the lungs and is often used to treat respiratory symptoms associated with colds and coughs, asthma, and bronchitis.

Geranium oil- is an essential oil often used to treat skin conditions such as bruises, burns, acne and eczema. It is also useful for treating insect related problems such as lice and can be used as a mosquito repellent.

Grapefruit oil- is an essential oil that is rich in vitamin C and so is great for boosting the immune system and treating colds. Because it helps remove excess water from the body it is often used to treat cellulite. It is also used to combat muscle fatigue and to encourage hair growth.

Green tea oil- is an essential oil often used for skin care due to it's anti-septic and anti-ageing properties.

Jasmine oil- is an essential oil which can be used to treat irritated or greasy skin. Other possible uses for jasmine oil include the treatment of depression and soothing of the nerves.

Juniper oil- is an essential oil often used to calm the nerves and relieve mental exhaustion.

Lavender oil- is a must have essential oil. It is often used to calm the nerves and to treat panic, depression and nervous exhaustion. It helps clear the airways and is used to treat bronchitis and asthma. Lavender can also help relieve muscle and joint pain associated with arthritis. For skin problems, lavender is useful for treating insect bites, stings and sunburn.

Lemon grass oil- is an essential oil which can be used for treating oily skin and acne. Lemon grass oil can also be used to relieve muscle pain and tone muscles.

Neroli oil- is an essential oil often used to treat shock, depression, anxiety and insomnia because of the calming effect it has. Because of its rejuvenating effects on skin, it can be used fight stretch marks and prevent scars.

Peppermint oil- is an essential oil which can be used to relieve itchy and irritated skin. It is also used to treat congestion of the sinuses and dry coughs. It should not be used around the eyes or by children or expectant mothers.

Rose oil- is an essential oil which can effectively be used to repair broken capillaries, as well as moisturise and hydrate the skin.

Rosemary oil- is an essential oil which is great for clearing the mind, improving memory and stimulating the brain because of its pronounced action on the nervous system and the brain. It is also for treating mental fatigue and headaches. It should not be used by people with high blood pressure or expectant mothers.

Sage oil- is an essential oil that can be used to treat depression as well as dermatitis, sores and ulcers. It can also be used to treat stiff or tired muscles. It should not be used by people with high blood pressure or expectant mothers.

Vanilla oil- is an essential oil which can be used to calm the mind and reduce anxiety.

Witch hazel oil- is an essential oil which can be used to treat bruising, sores, psoriasis and eczema.

Yarrow oil- is an essential oil which can be used as a mild anti-septic and to treat mild inflammation. Prolonged use may cause headaches and it should not be used by expectant mothers.